THE ULTIMATE DIABETES HACK

The Innovative Strategies to Master Diabetes Care, Revolutionise your Health and Feel Awesome While Moderating your Blood Sugar.

By

ELLIOT GORDON

TABLE OF CONTENT

CHAPTER ONE

CHAPTER TWO

CHAPTER THREE

CHAPTER SEVEN
CONCLUSION AND WORDS OF INSPIRATION.

Food is defined as any thing taken in order to offer energy or nutritive support to a living organism. Food is frequently deduced from shops or creatures and contains vital nutrients similar to carbs, lipids, proteins, vitamins, and minerals. Man has been nourished by food from the morning of time. Man has no way gone for an extended period of time without food. Food has was since the dawn of time. All shops and creatures bear nutrients to grow. The material is consumed by an organism and incorporated by its cells in order to give energy, sustain life, or stimulate growth. An essential nutrient is one that the body can not synthesize on its own — or not in sufficient quantities and must gain from the diet. These nutrients are needed for the body to serve duly, and they each support

7

different fleshly functions. Carbohydrates, protein, fat, vitamins, minerals, and water are the six necessary nutrients, and each can be set up in multitudinous factors of your diet.General nutritive information includes the main food groups needed to support the mortal body. Carbohydrates, which are necessary for energy, are set up in grains, fruits, and vegetables. Proteins, which are necessary for towel form and growth, are abundant in flesh, sap, and dairy products. Fats, which are necessary for numerous body conditioning, can be set up in canvases, nuts, and adipose fish. Vitamins and minerals included in a variety of diets promote general heartiness. Balance in these orders improves nutrition and promotes well- being. Understanding portion sizes and nutritive value can help you produce a well- balanced diet. Understanding these food groups lays the

8

root for making informed salutary opinions and living a healthier life.

These vital nutrients will be explained further below.

CARBOHYDRATES

Carbohydrates are the body's primary energy source, essential for powering different physiological systems and maintaining diurnal exertion. These macronutrients, which may be set up in a variety of foods similar as grains, fruits, and vegetables, come in a variety of forms, including simple sugars and complex carbs. Simple sugars, which are set up in reflections similar to fruits and reused sugars, give immediate energy boosts. Complex carbs, set up in whole grains, legumes, and stiff vegetables, on the other hand, give sustained energy and necessary salutary fibre, easing digestion and creating a sensation of wholeness. Choosing whole grain carbs over refined carbohydrates offers a slower release of energy and delivers critical rudiments that are generally removed from refined products. Carbohydrates in fibre not only regulate blood sugar situations but also promote digestive health, contributing to general well- being. It's critical to maintain a healthy carbohydrate input. While carbohydrates are an important source of energy, inordinate consumption, particularly of refined and reused carbs, can lead to weight gain and blood sugar swings. Including a variety of carbohydrates from nature's various palette provides a wide range of nutrients and health advantages. Understanding the differences between carbohydrate sources enables people to make further informed salutary choices, allowing them to harness the power of carbs for long- term vitality and general heartiness. Carbohydrates, the body's major source of energy, power our diurnal conditioning. They're abundant in grains, fruits, and vegetables and give both simple sugars and complex carbs for prolonged vitality. still, not all carbohydrates are created likewise; choosing whole grains versus refined choices guarantees a harmonious energy release as well as acceptable fibre for digestive health. Carbohydrate input must be balanced; inordinate consumption can contribute to weight gain and blood sugar swings. Embrace nature's various wealth to harness the power of carbs for long- term vigor and general heartiness. Carbohydrates are the body's primary energy source, essential for powering different physiological systems and maintaining diurnal exertion. These

11

macronutrients, which may be set up in a variety of foods similar as grains, fruits, and vegetables, come in a variety of forms, including simple sugars and complex carbs. Simple sugars, which are set up in refections similar as fruits and reused sugars, give immediate energy boosts. Complex carbs, set up in whole grains, legumes, and stiff vegetables, on the other hand, give sustained energy and necessary salutary fiber, easing digestion and creating a sensation of wholeness. Choosing whole grain carbs over refined carbohydrates offers a slower release of energy and delivers critical rudiments that are generally removed from refined products. Carbohydrates in fiber not only regulate blood sugar situations but also promote digestive health, contributing to general well- being. It's critical to maintain a healthy carbohydrate input. While carbohydrates are an important source of energy, inordinate consumption, particularly of refined and reused carbs, can lead to weight gain and blood sugar swings. Including a variety of carbohydrates from nature's various palette provides a wide range of nutrients and health advantages. Understanding the differences between carbohydrate sources enables people to make informed salutary choices, allowing them to harness the power of carbohydrates for long- term vitality and overall well- being.

PROTEINS

Proteins, the structure blocks of life, are critical macronutrients needed for towel form, vulnerable function support, and the facilitation of several metabolic conditioning within the body. These essential chemicals can be set up in a variety of foods, including flesh, flesh, fish, eggs, dairy, legumes, nuts, andseeds.Proteins, which are made up of amino acids, are divided into two types essential and unnecessary. The body can not synthesise essential amino acids and must admit them through salutary sources, emphasising the significance of a varied proteinconsumption.Complete   proteins containing all essential amino acids are set up in meat, fish, and dairy products. Factory- grounded sources,   similar as legumes, nuts, and seeds, give inadequate protein, demanding a combination of these refections to maintain a complete amino acidprofile.Protein consumption must be balanced for general health. While proteins are necessary for numerous introductory conditioning,   inordinate ingestion can strain renal function and beget other health

14

problems. A sufficient and different protein diet, on the other hand, promotes muscle conservation, aids in weight operation by adding malnutrition, and contributes to general well-being.Understanding the significance of proteins, their numerous sources, and the need of balance enables individualities to make informed salutary choices, allowing them to reap the advantages of proteins for optimal health and vitality.

FAT AND OIL

Fats and canvases are essential nutrients for our bodies. They give us energy and give essential adipose acids that we bear to stay healthy. Fats can be set up in canvases , nuts, seafood, and dairy products.

15

There are   colorful types of fats. Some, similar to those set up in beast products and some shops, can be dangerous to our hearts if consumed in excess. Others, similar as those set up in olive oil painting, almonds, and seafood, are salutary to our hearts. These nutritional fats can help keep our heart healthy.It's critical not to consume too important fat. Eating enough healthy fats helps us feel full, absorb vitamins, and keep   our   bodies   running   easily. Understanding which fats are salutary and how   important to consume allows us to make healthier eating choices.

VITAMINS

These are chemical motes that our bodies bear in little quantities for a variety of critical tasks. There are two types of vitamins fat-answerable vitamins(A, D, E, and K) and water-answerable vitamins(B-complex and vitamin C). - Fat-answerable vitamins are stored in the adipose apkins and liver of the body. Vitamin A is necessary for healthy vision, immunological function, and cell growth. Vitamin D aids calcium immersion, which is necessary for strong bones and teeth. Vitamin E functions as an antioxidant, precluding cell damage. Vitamin K is needed for proper blood coagulation and bone health. - Water-answerable vitamins dissolve in water and aren't kept in considerable amounts in the body, with the exception of B12, which can be stored in the liver. Vitamin C and B-complex vitamins(B1, B2, B3, B5, B6, B7, B9, and B12) help in energy product, metabolism, whim-whams function, red blood cell creation, and maintaining healthy skin, hair, and eyes.

17

Each vitamin has its own nutritive source. Vitamin A, for illustration, is generous in liver, carrots, and spinach, whereas vitamin C is current in citrus fruits and vegetables. scarcities in particular vitamins can beget a variety of health problems, similar as night blindness due to a lack of vitamin A or scurvy due to a lack of vitaminC. A well-balanced diet rich in fruits, vegetables, whole grains, spare flesh, and dairy products generally provides an applicable force of important vitamins. Supplements may be advised in some situations, particularly for people with specific salutary restrictions or medical issues. Before beginning any supplements plan, always consult with a healthcare expert.

MINERAL SALT

Mineral salts are classified as"non-energetic nutrients," or important minerals for our bodies that don't give energy or calories. Mineral mariners can be set up in food and must be incorporated into a   diurnal nutrition that's varied and full in order to insure the optimal input of this vast class of nutrients. A monotonous diet clearly lacks integration each dish stands out for its sweet quantum, energetic nutritive composition(carbohydrates, lipids, and proteins), and non-energetic nutrients similar as mineral mariners.   Sodium, chlorine, potassium, magnesium, calcium, phosphorus, and iron are the most vital minerals for   mortal bodies, and their consumption should be balanced. Because of the important places that they perform, the damage from both redundant and disfigurement is known.

WATER

Water is necessary for the majority of body activities.
The body has no mechanism of storing water and requires fresh supplies every day.
The finest source of fluids is fresh tap water.
Depending on their age and gender, a child will require varying amounts of fluid.
Women should drink about 2 litres (8 cups) of fluids per day, while males should drink about 2.6 litres (10 cups).
People who are pregnant or breastfeeding require more fluids per day than usual.
Dehydration can occur when the body's fluids are depleted. It can be fatal, especially to babies, children, and the elderly. But it's just been a few days without water.

The human body is 50 to 75% water. Water is the primary component of blood, digestive fluids, urine, and perspiration, as well as lean muscle, fat, and bones.

Because the body cannot store water, we require fresh supplies every day to compensate for losses from the lungs, skin, urine, and faeces (poo). The amount we require is determined by our body size, metabolism, the weather, the foods we eat, and our degree of exercise.

Water facts include:

Body water content is higher in men than in women, and it decreases with age in both.

Most mature adults lose 2.5 to 3 litres of water every day. Water loss may increase in hot temperatures and with extended exertion.

The elderly lose roughly 2 litres every day.

21

A three-hour flight can cause a person to lose around 1.5 litres of water.

Water loss must be restored.

WATER'S IMPORTANCE -Water is required for most bodily activities, including:

-Keep every cell in the body healthy and intact.

-Keep the circulation liquid enough to move through blood vessels.

-Aid in the elimination of metabolic byproducts, excess electrolytes (such as sodium and potassium), and urea, a waste product generated during the digestion of dietary protein.

-Sweating helps to regulate body temperature.

-Moist mucous membranes (such as those in the lungs and mouth).

-Lubricate and cushion joints.

-Reduce the risk of urinary tract infections (UTIs), such as cystitis, by keeping the bladder free of microorganisms.
Aid digestion and prevent constipation.
-Moisturise the skin to keep its texture and appearance.
-Carry nutrients and oxygen to cells.
-Act as a shock absorber inside the eyes, spinal cord, and the amniotic sac enclosing the foetus during pregnancy.

Water in our food

Most meals, including ones that appear hard and dry, contain water. Solid foods alone can provide roughly 20% of the body's overall water requirements.

As a byproduct of the digestion process, the body receives a little amount of water. Water obtained in this manner can meet around 10% of the body's water requirements.

The remaining 70% or so of water necessary by the body must come from fluids (liquids).

CHAPTER TWO

UNDERSTANDING DIABETES

WHAT IS DIABETES

Diabetes is a condition that develops when your blood glucose, frequently known as blood sugar, is abnormally high. Glucose is the primary source of energy in your body. Although your body can produce glucose, it also obtains glucose from the food you consume. Insulin is a hormone produced by the pancreas that aids in the transport of glucose into cells for use as energy. Diabetes occurs when your body doesn't produce enough — or any — insulin or doesn't use insulin meetly. Glucose therefore remains in your rotation rather than reaching your cells. Diabetes increases the threat of eye, order, whim-whams, and heart problems. Diabetes has also been connected to certain types of cancer. Taking conduct to avoid or manage diabetes may reduce your chances of getting diabetes- related health issues. Diabetes mellitus is a metabolic complaint characterised by elevated blood sugar situations. Your body either doesn't produce enough insulin or doesn't use the insulin that it does produce adequately.   Insulin transports sugar from the blood into your cells, where it's stored or used for energy.However, you may have diabetes, If

25

this fails. Diabetes- related elevated blood sugar can harm your jitters, eyes, feathers, and other organs if left undressed. Still, learning about diabetes and taking sweats to help or control it can help guard your health.

TYPES OF DIABETES

1. TYPE 1 DIABETES

Type 1 diabetes occurs when your body produces little or no insulin. Your immune system targets and destroys insulin-producing cells in your pancreas. Type 1 diabetes is most commonly diagnosed in children and young adults, but it can occur at any age. To stay alive, people with type 1 diabetes must take insulin every day. Type 1 diabetes develops when the immune system erroneously assaults and destroys the pancreas' insulin-producing cells (beta cells). As a result, the body produces insufficient insulin, resulting in an excess of glucose in the bloodstream.

2.TYPE 2 DIABETES:

Type 2 diabetes occurs when the cells in your body do not effectively use insulin. The pancreas may produce insulin, but not enough to keep your blood glucose levels within the usual range. The most frequent type of diabetes is type 2. If you have risk factors for type 2 diabetes, such as being overweight or obese, as well as a family history of the condition, you are more likely to develop it. Type 2 diabetes can strike at any age, including youth.

27

Knowing the risk factors for type 2 diabetes and adopting efforts towards a better lifestyle, such as decreasing weight or limiting weight gain, can help delay or prevent the disease.The body grows resistant to the effects of insulin or does not produce enough insulin to sustain normal glucose levels in this kind. It is frequently associated with lifestyle variables such as obesity, physical inactivity, and hereditary predisposition.

DIFFERENCES BETWEEN TYPE 1 AND TYPE 2 DIABETES.

If you have type 1 or type 2 diabetes, it means you have an excess of glucose (a form of sugar) in your blood owing to an issue with the hormone insulin. Both are significant conditions with serious health consequences. However, the aetiology, onset of symptoms, and treatment of type 1 and type 2 diabetes differ.

When you have type 1 diabetes, your body is unable to produce any insulin. Your immune system has attacked and killed the insulin-producing cells. This is why type 1 diabetes is referred to as an autoimmune disease.

Type 2 diabetes is not an autoimmune disease. Your body isn't producing enough insulin, or what it is producing isn't working effectively. This could be for a variety of reasons.

Type 1 diabetes represents 8% of those with diabetes, while type 2 diabetes affects 90% of those with diabetes. There are also additional forms of diabetes.

You need information, treatment, and support to manage your diabetes, regardless of the type.

Differences between types 1 and 2

The table below summarizes some of the key distinctions between type 1 and type 2.

	Type 1	Type 2
Causes	Your body attacks the cells in your pancreas which means it cannot	Your body is unable to make enough insulin or the insulin you do make doesn't

	make any insulin.	work properly.
Risk factors	We don't yet know what causes type 1 diabetes. Family history can slightly increase your risk, as there are a number of genes	Your age, family history, ethnicity, your waist circumference and living with obesity or overweight are all risk factors for

	linked to type 1 diabetes.	type 2 diabetes.
Symptoms	The symptoms for type 1 appear more quickly.	Symptoms for type 2 diabetes can be easier to miss because they appear more slowly. And you may not notice

		any symptoms.
Management	You treat type 1 by taking insulin. You count the carbohydrates you eat and drink and try to balance	Unlike type 1 diabetes, sometimes type 2 diabetes can be treated without taking insulin or other medication to help

this with doses of insulin.

Being as active as possible, eating healthily and going for regular health checks is also important.

lower your blood sugar levels. Getting support to being as active as possible, eating healthily and going for regular health checks can help you manage it.

Cure and Prevention

Currently there is no cure for type 1 but research continues. We could speak of management

Type 2 cannot be cured but there is evidence to say in many cases it can be prevented and put into remission.

*3.*GESTATIONAL DIABETES:

Diabetes that develops during pregnancy is known as gestational diabetes. This type of diabetes usually goes away once the baby is born. However, if you have experienced gestational diabetes, you are more likely to develop type 2 diabetes later in life. Type 2 diabetes is sometimes diagnosed during pregnancy.

GENERAL SYMPTOMS OF DIABETES

FREQUENT URINATION: Excess sugar in the blood encourages the kidneys to work harder to filter and absorb the excess sugar. This causes increased urine as the body attempts to remove the extra glucose.

37

FREQUENT THIRST: Frequent urine can cause dehydration, causing a person to feel excessively thirsty and drink extra fluids to compensate for fluid loss.

EXTREME HUNGER: When cells become insulin resistant (as in type 2 diabetes) or when there is a lack of insulin (as in type 1 diabetes), glucose cannot enter the cells to provide energy. This can lead to prolonged hunger even after eating.

UNEXPLAINED WEIGHT LOSS: When the body is unable to correctly use glucose, it may begin breaking down muscle tissue and fat for energy, resulting in unintended weight loss.

EXHAUSTION: When there is insufficient glucose entering the cells to provide energy, exhaustion and weakness can arise as the body attempts to function efficiently.

BLURRY VISION: High blood sugar levels can cause the lens of the eye to expand, impairing the ability to concentrate and resulting in blurred vision.

SLOW HEALING SCORES: High blood sugar levels can impair the body's ability to heal, resulting in slower healing of wounds and sores.

INFECTIONS: High blood sugar levels can weaken the immune system, making the body more prone to infections and slowing the healing process.

TINGLING OR NUMBNESS: High blood sugar levels can cause nerve damage, resulting in tingling, numbness, or even pain in the hands and feet (diabetic neuropathy). Dry, itchy skin: High blood sugar levels can cause skin dryness and itching, causing discomfort.

YEAST INFECTIONS: Increased glucose levels in vaginal secretions can produce a more conducive environment for yeast to

39

thrive, leading to more frequent yeast infections in women.

IRRITABILITY: Changes in blood sugar levels can influence mood and cause irritability or mood swings.

Remember that the intensity of these symptoms might vary and that they do not always indicate diabetes. If you have any of these symptoms, you should see a doctor for an accurate evaluation and diagnosis.

SOME IMPORTANT FACTORS IN THE DEVELOPMENT OF DIABETES.

Several factors influence diabetes development:
- genetics
- Diet
- Lifestyle choices

40

- Physical activity
- Obesity
- Ethnicity, age, and family history are all environmental influences.

These factors frequently interact, increasing the risk and progression of diabetes.

CHAPTER THREE

UNDERSTANDING YOUR BLOOD GLUCOSE (SUGAR) LEVEL

TEST FOR GLUCOSE (SUGAR) IN THE BLOOD

A blood glucose test determines the quantum of glucose(sugar) in your blood. The test may number a galette burrow or a blood sample from a tone. Blood glucose testing are the most regularly used system by healthcare interpreters to screen for Type 2 diabetes, which is a common disorder.What exactly is a blood glucose(sugar) test? A blood glucose test is a blood test that primarily defends diabetes by measuring the position of glucose(sugar) in your blood.

TYPES OF BLOOD SUGAR TESTS

Capillary blood glucose test:A healthcare expert collects a drop of blood, generally from a fingertip burrow. These tests use a test strip and a glucose metre(glucometer), which indicate your blood sugar position in seconds.

Venous(tube) blood glucose test: A phlebotomist draws blood from a tone(venipuncture). These glucose tests are generally part of a blood panel, similar as a introductory metabolic panel. The samples will be transferred to a laboratory by the provider. A medical laboratory scientist will prepare your samples and do the tests on analyzers. Venous blood glucose testing is constantly more accurate than capillary blood glucose tests. Gobbling blood glucose tests are constantly ordered by croakers to screen for diabetes. Because eating refections influences blood sugar, gorging blood glucose tests give a more accurate picture of your birth blood sugar. For diabetics, there's also at- home blood sugar testing(using a glucometer). People with Type 1 diabetes, in particular, must test their blood sugar situations multitudinous times per day in order to effectively manage the

44

condition.   Nonstop glucose monitoring bias(CGMs) are another possibility. Several natural mechanisms work together to keep your blood glucose situations in a healthy range. Insulin, a hormone produced by the pancreas, is the most important factor in maintaining normal blood sugar situations. Hyperglycemia(high blood glucose situations) constantly suggests diabetes. Diabetes occurs when your pancreas fails to produce enough insulin or when your body fails to respond correctly to the goods of insulin.

WHAT IS BLOOD SUGAR?

Glucose(sugar) is substantially deduced from carbs set up in food and potables. It's your body's primary source of energy. Your blood transports glucose to all of your body's cells for use as energy. Several natural mechanisms work together to keep your blood glucose situations in a healthy range. Insulin, a hormone produced by the pancreas, is the most important factor in maintaining normal blood sugar situations. Hyperglycemia(high blood glucose situations) constantly suggests diabetes. Diabetes occurs when your pancreas fails to produce enough insulin or when your body fails to respond correctly to the goods of insulin.

WHEN AND WHY WOULD I NEED A BLOOD GLUCOSE TEST?

There are three primary motivations behind why you might require a blood glucose (sugar) test:

 Your medical services supplier might have requested routine blood work called a fundamental metabolic board (BMP) or an exhaustive metabolic board (CMP), which both incorporate a glucose blood test.

You might be having side effects of high glucose or low glucose, which could show diabetes or another condition.

On the off chance that you take a drawn out prescription that influences your glucose levels, for example, corticosteroids, you might require routine glucose blood tests to screen your levels.

The most widely recognized utilization of a blood glucose test is to evaluate for Type 2 diabetes (T2D), which is a typical condition. Certain individuals are in danger of creating Type 2 diabetes. Assuming you have risk factors, your supplier will probably suggest customary screening regardless of your age. The American Diabetes Affiliation suggests customary evaluating for anybody age 35 or more established.

Your supplier will likewise arrange a blood glucose test on the off chance that you have side effects of high glucose (hyperglycemia) or low glucose (hypoglycemia).

Side effects of diabetes and high glucose level include:

- Feeling exceptionally parched (polydipsia).
- Regular pee (polyuria).

- Weariness.
- Feeling exceptionally eager (polyphagia).
- Unexplained weight reduction.

- Obscured vision.
- Slow mending of cuts or wounds.

In the event that you or your kid have these side effects as well as heaving, profound work breathing or potentially disarray, go to the closest trauma center at the earliest opportunity. You might have diabetes-related ketoacidosis, which is a perilous condition.

Side effects of low glucose level include:

- Shaking or shudder.
- Perspiring and chills.
- Discombobulation or dizziness.
- Quicker pulse.

- Profound appetite.
- Nervousness or crabbiness.

You really want to drink carbs (sugar) to treat hypoglycemia, like a banana or squeezed apple. Serious hypoglycemia can life-compromise.

WHO PERFORMS A BLOOD GLUCOSE TEST

Numerous medical care suppliers, like medical attendants, can play out a hairlike (finger prick) blood glucose test. These tests include a glucose meter and a test strip, which show your glucose result in practically no time.

Phlebotomists commonly perform venous blood glucose tests. They send the examples to a lab for testing.

HOW WOULD I PREPARE FOR A BLOOD GLUCOSE TEST

On the off chance that your medical services supplier has requested a fasting blood glucose test, you'll have to not eat or drink anything with the exception of water (quick) for eight to 10 hours before the test.

In the event that your blood glucose test is important for a fundamental or exhaustive metabolic board, you may likewise have to quick for a few hours before your blood draw. Regardless, your medical services supplier will inform you as to whether you want to adhere to any extraordinary directions.

WHAT DO I EXPECT DURING A BLOOD GLUCOSE TEST

53

You can expect the accompanying during a venous glucose test, or blood draw:

You'll sit in a seat, and a phlebotomist will really look at your arms for an effectively open vein. This is as a rule in the internal piece of your arm on the opposite side of your elbow. Whenever they've found a vein, they'll clean and sanitize the region.

.WHAT DO THE RESULTS OF A GLUCOSE TEST MEAN?

Blood test reports, including blood glucose test reports, generally give the accompanying data The name of the blood test or what was estimated in your blood. The number or estimation of your blood test result. The typical estimation range for that test. Data that shows assuming your outgrowth is typical or unusual or high or low.

WHAT'S NORMAL GLUCOSE LEVEL IN THE BLOOD

A solid(typical) fasting blood glucose position for notoriety without diabetes is 70 to 99 mg/ dL(3.9 to5.5 mmol/ L). Values nearly in the range of 50 and 70 mg/ dL(2.8 to3.9 mmol/ L) for individuals without diabetes can be" ordinary" as well.

WHAT DOES HIGH GLUCOSE LEVEL MEAN

On the off chance that your fasting blood glucose position is 100 to 125 mg/ dL(5.6 to 6.9 mmol/ L), it as a rule implies you have prediabetes. individuals with prediabetes have up to a half possibility of creating Type 2 diabetes throughout the following five to 10 times. Yet, you can do whatever it may take to keep Type 2 diabetes from creating. In the event that your fasting blood glucose position is 126 mg/ dl(7.0 mmol/ L) or advanced further than one testing event, it as a rule implies you have diabetes. In both of these cases, your supplier will presumably arrange a glycated hemoglobin test(A1c) prior to diagnosing you with prediabetes or diabetes. An A1c shows your typical glucose further than a couple of months.

CHAPTER FOUR

UNDERSTANDING PRE DIABETES

Prediabetes is defined as having blood sugar situations that are more advanced than normal. It isn't yet high enough to be classified as type 2 diabetes. Grown-ups and children with prediabetes are at significant threat of developing type 2 diabetes if no life variations are made. Still, the long- term damage caused by diabetes, particularly to your heart, If you have prediabetes. Still, there's some good news. The progression from prediabetes to class 2 diabetes isn't automatic. Eating healthy foods, incorporating physical exertion into your diurnal routine, and maintaining a healthy weight can all help to restore your blood sugar situations to normal. The same life adaptations that can help avoid type 2 diabetes in grown-ups may also help restore normal blood sugar situations in youths.

PREDIABETES SIGNS AND SYMPTOMS Prediabetes typically has no suggestions or symptoms. Darkened skin on some regions of the body is one probable symptom of prediabetes. The neck, armpits, and groin can all be affected. The following signs and symptoms indicate that you have progressed from pre-diabetes to Type 2 diabetes

- jacked thirst
- Urination on a regular base
- heightened hunger
- Fatigue
- Vision deformation
- bottom or hand impassiveness
- Blisters that take a long time to heal

- Unintentional weight loss

WHAT EXACTLY ARE THE CAUSES OF PREDIABETES?

It's unknown what causes prediabetes. Still, family history and genetics appear to play a significant effect. What's apparent is that persons with prediabetes no longer adequately digest sugar(glucose). The maturity of the glucose in your body is deduced from the food you eat. Sugar enters your bloodstream during digestion. Insulin lets sugar into your cells while dwindling the volume of sugar in your blood. The pancreas, a gland set up behind the stomach, produces insulin.

When you eat, your pancreas releases insulin into your bloodstream. When your blood sugar situations begin to fall, the pancreas limits the release of insulin into the blood. When you have prediabetes, this medium is bloodied. As a result, rather than feeding your cells, sugar accumulates in your bloodstream. This is possible because Your pancreas may be producing inadequate insulin. Your cells come insulin resistant and allow lower sugar into your body. threat rudiments The same factors that raise the liability of developing type 2 diabetes also increase the liability of developing prediabetes. These rudiments are as follows Weight. rotundity is a major threat factor for prediabetes. The further adipose towel you have, particularly outside and between the muscle and skin girding your tummy, the further insulin resistant your cells come. Waist circumference. Insulin resistance might be indicated by a big midriff size. Men with middles larger than 40 elevation and women with middles larger than 35 elevation are more likely to develop insulin resistance. Diet. Consuming red and reused meat, as well as drinking sugar- candied potables, has been linked to an increased threat of prediabetes. Inactivity. The less active you are, the more likely you're to get prediabetes. Age. Although diabetes can occur at any age, the threat of prediabetes rises after the age of 35.

A familytree.However, you're more likely to develop prediabetes, If you have a parent or stock who has type 2 diabetes.

A person's race or race. Although it's unknown why, certain ethnical groups, similar as Black, Hispanic, American Indian, and Asian Americans, are more likely to acquire prediabetes.

Diabetes during gestation. You and your child are more likely to develop prediabetes if you had diabetes while pregnant(gravid diabetes). Polycystic ovarian pattern(PCOS). Women who have this common complaint, which is characterised by irregular menstrual cycles, inordinate hair growth, and rotundity, are at an increased threat of developing prediabetes.

Sleep. Insulin resistance is more common in people who have obstructive sleep apnea, a complaint that disturbs sleep regularly. fat or fat people are more likely to develop obstructive sleep apnea.

Tobacco use. Smoking may raise insulin resistance and increase the chance of type 2 diabetes in those with prediabetes, as well as the threat of diabetic complications.

The following are 12 steps that may see in the reversal of prediabetes:

- Focus on a well-balanced diet that includes plenty of vegetables, fruits, whole grains, lean proteins, and healthy fats. Limit your intake of sugar, refined carbohydrates, and processed meals.

- **Regular Exercise**: Be physically active on most days of the week. Aim for 150 minutes per week of moderate exercise, such as brisk walking or cycling.

- **Weight Loss**: Even a small amount of weight loss can greatly increase insulin sensitivity and lessen the chance of developing diabetes.

- **Portion regulation**: Pay attention to portion sizes to avoid overeating and to limit calorie intake, which can help with weight loss and blood sugar regulation.

- Drink plenty of water throughout the day to stay hydrated and improve your overall health.

- **Monitor Blood Sugar:** Check your blood sugar levels on a regular basis, as directed by your healthcare physician, to track changes and evaluate the effectiveness of lifestyle adjustments.

- **Stress Reduction:** Because stress can affect blood sugar levels, try stress-reduction practices such as meditation, yoga, or deep breathing exercises.

- **Adequate Sleep:** Get adequate quality sleep each night because lack of sleep might alter blood sugar levels and insulin sensitivity.

- Reduce or eliminate alcohol consumption because it might influence blood sugar levels and contribute to weight gain.

- Schedule regular check-ups with your healthcare provider to track progress, alter methods, and verify you're on track to reverse prediabetes.

- **Foods High in Fibre:** Consume additional fibre in your diet by eating beans, lentils, whole grains, and fruits. Fibre improves fullness and helps with blood sugar regulation.

- **Behavioural adjustments:** Rather than relying on fast fixes, adopt healthy habits for the long term by implementing gradual, sustainable lifestyle adjustments. The key to reversing prediabetes is consistency.

CHAPTER FIVE

MANAGEMENT PLAN FOR DIABETES.

Diabetes management necessitates education. Understand what causes your blood sugar levels to rise and fall — and how to manage these day-to-day issues.

When diet and exercise are insufficient for treating diabetes, insulin and other diabetes medicines are used to lower blood sugar levels. The success of these drugs, however, is dependent on the time and size of the dose. Medications taken for diseases other than diabetes can potentially have an impact on your blood sugar levels.

MEDICATION AND INSULIN THERAPY

Medication and insulin therapy are critical components of diabetes management. Metformin, sulfonylureas, SGLT-2 inhibitors, and other medications assist manage blood sugar levels. Insulin therapy is required for type 1 diabetes and is occasionally required for type 2 diabetes when other drugs are insufficient. It aids in glucose regulation by replicating the body's normal insulin production or supplementing when the body does not create enough. Individuals with diabetes must collaborate closely with healthcare specialists to identify the best effective treatment plan.

What you should do:

Insulin should be stored correctly. Insulin that has been incorrectly stored or has passed its expiration date may no longer be effective. Insulin is particularly sensitive to temperature fluctuations.

Inform your doctor about any issues. If your diabetes drugs cause your blood sugar to dip too low or rise too high on a regular basis, the dosage or timing may need to be modified.

Be wary of new drugs. If you are thinking about taking an over-the-counter medicine or if your doctor recommends a new medication to address another illness, such as high blood pressure or high cholesterol, ask your doctor or chemist if the medication will affect your blood sugar levels.

A different drug may be prescribed in some cases. Always with your doctor before starting any new over-the-counter medicine so you understand how it will affect your blood sugar level.

EXERCISE AND PHYSICAL ACTIVITIES' ROLE

Physical activity is another critical component of your diabetes control strategy. When you exercise, your muscles generate energy from sugar (glucose). Regular physical activity also aids your body's usage of insulin.

These elements work together to reduce your blood sugar level. The longer the effect lasts, the more strenuous your workout. However, even simple activities like housework, gardening, or standing for long periods of time might help your blood sugar.

What you should do:

Consult your doctor about an activity programme. Consult your doctor about the best sort of exercise for you. In general, most individuals should engage in at least 150 minutes of moderate aerobic activity every week. On most days of the week, aim for 30 minutes of moderate aerobic activity.

If you've been inactive for a long time, your doctor may want to assess your general health before making a recommendation. He or she can advise on the best combination of aerobic and muscle-strengthening activity.

Maintain a regular exercise routine. Consult your doctor about the optimal time of day to exercise so that your workout programme coincides with your meal and prescription routines.

Understand your numbers. Before you begin exercising, consult with your doctor about what blood sugar levels are appropriate for you.

Examine your blood sugar levels. Check your blood sugar levels before, during, and after exercise, especially if you take insulin or blood sugar-lowering drugs. Exercise can drop your blood sugar levels even up to a day later, especially if you're doing it for the first time or at a higher intensity. Be mindful of symptoms of low blood sugar, such as shakiness, weakness, fatigue, hunger, lightheadedness, irritability, anxiety, or confusion.

If you use insulin and your blood sugar level is less than 90 milligrammes per deciliter (mg/dL) or 5.0 millimoles per litre (mmol/L), eat a little snack before you begin exercising to avoid hypoglycemia.

Keep hydrated. While exercising, drink plenty of water or other fluids because dehydration might alter blood sugar levels.

Prepare yourself. Carry a small snack or glucose tablets with you when exercising in case your blood sugar gets too low. Wear a medical identification bracelet at all times.

As needed, modify your diabetes treatment strategy. If you use insulin, you may need to lower your insulin dose before exercising and closely monitor your blood sugar for several hours after strenuous exercise since delayed hypoglycemia can occur. Your doctor can advise you on proper drug modifications. If you've increased your workout habit, you may need to modify your treatment.

THE IMPACT OF NUTRITION AND DIET

Healthy nutrition is an essential component of living a healthy lifestyle, whether you have diabetes or not. However, if you have diabetes, you must understand how foods affect your blood sugar levels. It is not only the sort of food you eat, but also how much you eat and how you combine different types of food.

What you should do:

Discover carbohydrate counting and portion sizes. Learning how to measure carbohydrates is an important part of many diabetes control strategies. Carbohydrates have the greatest impact on blood sugar levels. It is critical for persons using mealtime insulin to understand the amount of carbohydrates in their diet so that they receive the correct insulin dose.

Discover the proper portion size for each meal type. Write down quantities for meals you eat frequently to simplify meal planning. To guarantee adequate portion size and an exact carbohydrate count, use measuring cups or a scale.

Make sure that every meal is well-balanced. Plan your meals to include a variety of grains, fruits and vegetables, proteins, and fats as much as possible. Pay attention to the carbohydrates you consume.

Some carbohydrates are better for you than others, such as fruits, vegetables, and whole grains. These foods are low in carbohydrates and high in fibre, which helps maintain blood sugar levels constant.

Consult your doctor, nurse, or nutritionist about the optimal dietary choices and the proper food type balance.

Plan your meals and medications. Too little meals in relation to your diabetes treatments, particularly insulin, can lead to dangerously low blood sugar levels (hypoglycemia). A high blood sugar level (hyperglycemia) can result from eating too much. Discuss how to effectively coordinate meal and medication schedules with your diabetes health care team.
Drinks with added sugar should be avoided. Sugar-sweetened beverages are heavy in calories and low in nutrients. If you have diabetes, you should avoid these drinks since they cause blood sugar to spike quickly.

The only exception is if you have a low blood sugar level. Sugar-sweetened beverages, such as soda, juice and sports drinks, can be used to swiftly raise blood sugar levels that are too low.

CHAPTER SIX

STAYING CONSISTENT IN THE STRIVE.

Consistency is essential in diabetes management. A balanced diet, frequent exercise, medication adherence, and blood sugar monitoring all help significantly.

You may be encouraged to undertake lifestyle adjustments to control type 2 diabetes. Your doctor may advise you to monitor your blood sugar levels on a regular basis. They may also give you oral drugs or other therapies.

You may feel overwhelmed by the quantity of adjustments you need to make, which is where goal-setting comes in.

Setting precise, measurable goals can aid in the development of healthy behaviours and the adherence to your treatment plan. Continue reading to learn about treatment goal-setting strategies.
Set goals that will encourage healthy habits. Keeping your blood sugar within a specific range reduces your risk of type 2 diabetes complications. Adopting healthy habits can assist you in reaching and maintaining your goal range.

Consider reflecting on your present lifestyle patterns and the changes you could make to better manage your illness.

You could, for example, gain from:

- modifying your eating habits
- .increasing your physical activity, sleeping more, minimizing stress, and monitoring your blood sugar levels more frequently
- taking your prescription meds on a regular basis
- Even minor modifications in your behaviours may have a favourable impact on your blood sugar levels or general health.

SET REALISTIC AND SPECIFIC GOALS

Setting a reasonable goal increases your chances of success. That success may inspire you to establish new goals and keep making progress over time.

It is also critical to identify clear goals. Setting precise goals allows you to know what you want to accomplish and when you've accomplished it. This may assist you in making concrete progress.

For example, "exercise more" is a reasonable goal, but it is not very detailed. A more precise objective may be to "go for a half-hour walk in the evening, five days a week for the next month."

Other specific objectives include:

"visit the gym on Mondays, Wednesdays, and Saturdays for the next month"
"cut my cookie consumption from three to one per day for the next two months"

"lose fifteen pounds over the next three months"

"try a new recipe from my diabetes cookbook every week"

"check my blood sugar levels two times a day for the next two weeks"

Consider what you want to accomplish, how you intend to accomplish it, and when you intend to accomplish it.

MONITOR YOUR PROGRESS

Consider keeping a notebook, a smartphone app, or other tools to track your progress towards your goals. This can help you stay on track over time.

Many apps, for example, are available for tracking calories and meals, gym sessions, and other activities. A basic checklist pinned to your refrigerator may be sufficient in some circumstances.

If you're having trouble reaching your goals, consider the obstacles you've encountered and develop solutions to overcome them. In some circumstances, you may need to modify a goal to make it more feasible.

After you've accomplished one goal, you can set another to build on your progress.

COLLABORATE WITH YOUR HEALTH CARE TEAM

Your healthcare team can assist you in setting and meeting type 2 diabetes management objectives.

Your doctor or nurse practitioner, for example, may recommend you to a qualified dietitian to establish a meal plan that meets your healthy eating or weight loss objectives. Alternatively, they may recommend you to a physical therapist to establish a safe workout plan for you.

A doctor or nurse practitioner can also assist you in determining an appropriate blood sugar target.

The A1C test will be used to track your blood sugar levels over time. This blood test measures your three-month average blood sugar levels.

According to the American Diabetes Association, an acceptable A1C target for many non-pregnant persons is less than 7% (53 mmol/mol).

However, your healthcare practitioner may advise you to set a target that is somewhat lower or higher in some situations.

They will consider your current condition and medical history while determining an appropriate aim.

BE COMPASSIONATE WITH YOURSELF AND CELEBRATE YOUR SUCCESSES.

If you're having trouble keeping your blood sugar within the target range or meeting other treatment goals, don't be too hard on yourself.

Even if you follow your suggested treatment plan, type 2 diabetes is a complex disorder that can vary over time.

Other life changes and problems can also make it difficult to reach your treatment objectives.

Inform your healthcare practitioner if you are having difficulty meeting your objectives.They may recommend adjustments to your lifestyle behaviours, prescribed drugs, or other aspects of your treatment plan in some situations. They may also make changes to your blood sugar aim over time.

Setting realistic and detailed goals may help you lower your blood sugar levels and lower your risk of type 2 diabetes problems. Your healthcare team can assist you in setting and achieving objectives that are appropriate for your situation.

Speak with your doctor about some of the goals you could make to assist manage your condition.

KEY FACTS ABOUT DIABETES

1.Type 2 diabetes affects the great majority of people worldwide.

2. Diabetes is the biggest cause of death worldwide. 3. Type 1 diabetes is more common in adolescents.

4.Type 2 diabetes is avoidable.

5. Diabetes can be well treated.

6. Diabetes meal preparation does not have to be difficult.

7. Diabetes is a leading cause of amputation, renal failure, and other health problems.

8. Knowing your risk level can help you plan for or avoid diabetes. 9. Having gestational diabetes does not guarantee that your child will have it.

10. Diabetes can elicit a wide range of feelings.

CHAPTER SEVEN

CONCLUSION AND WORDS OF INSPIRATION.

Diabetes can be a difficult road, but it's vital to realise that you're stronger than you believe. Diabetes management is about more than simply blood sugar levels; it's about perseverance, determination, and a dedication to your health.

Every day, you must maintain a delicate balance of medication, nutrition, exercise, and monitoring, which requires tremendous strength. It's okay to feel frustrated or exhausted at times, but never lose sight of the courage required to fight this disease head on.

Remember that having diabetes does not define you. It is a part of your life, but it does not decrease or limit your worth. You are capable of extraordinary things, and your diabetes path demonstrates your perseverance and flexibility.

Seek assistance from loved ones, medical professionals, and support organisations. Sharing your experiences, struggles, and triumphs can help to lighten the load while also providing vital insights and encouragement. You are not alone on this path, and there is a community waiting to pull you up and empower you.

Celebrate your accomplishments, no matter how minor they appear to be. Every blood sugar check, every healthy meal choice, and every minute of physical exercise is a step towards a healthier you. Accept your triumphs and use them as inspiration to keep going.

Exercise self-compassion. Living with diabetes can be difficult, and it's normal to experience setbacks. Kindness and understanding should be extended to yourself. Learn from your mistakes and use them to help you develop and improve.

Learn everything you can about diabetes. Knowledge gives you power. Understanding how your body works, how different foods and activities influence you, and being up to date on diabetes treatment advances can provide you with a sense of control and confidence.

Find hobbies that make you happy and help you deal with stress. Prioritising your mental well-being, whether through art, reading, yoga, or spending time in nature, is critical in effectively managing diabetes.

Remember that self-care is not selfish; it is vital. Prioritise self-care. Get enough sleep, practice mindfulness, and schedule things that will revitalize your spirit.

Finally, never give up hope. Every day, science and medicine advance. On the horizon are continuous studies, new technology, and improved treatments. Your fortitude and resolve will see you through, and better days are on the way.

95

Diabetes does not define you. You are powerful, capable, and tenacious. Continue to believe in yourself, strive for improved health, and embrace the adventure with courage and commitment. You've got this.